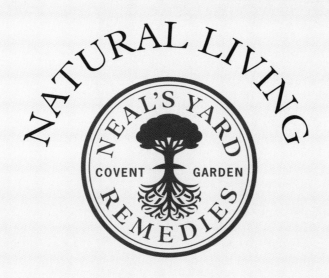

NATURAL LIVING

NEAL'S YARD
COVENT GARDEN
REMEDIES

DETOX

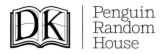

Editors Susannah Steel, Sarah Ruddick,
Libby Brown
Designers Alison Gardner, Kathryn Wilding
Jacket Designer Vanessa Hamilton
Producer, Pre-Production Rebecca Fallowfield
Production Controller Isobel Reid
Special Sales Creative Project Manager
Alison Donovan

Content previously published in *Neal's Yard Remedies*
(2011) by Dorling Kindersley Limited
80 Strand, London, WC2R 0RL

2 4 6 8 10 9 7 5 3 1
001 – 309660 – Dec/2017

ISBN 978-0-2413-3404-1

Printed and bound in China

A WORLD OF IDEAS
SEE ALL THERE IS TO KNOW
www.dk.com

DISCLAIMER: See page 48

CONTENTS

Juices and smoothies **4**

Teas **14**

Tinctures **18**

Soups **22**

Salads **28**

Body creams **32**

Cleansers **34**

Face masks **38**

Bath infusions **42**

Hair and scalp treatments **46**

Acknowledgments **48**

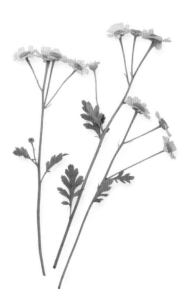

INTRODUCTION

According to the World Health Organization, herbal remedies are the most widespread system of medicine used in the world. In many developed countries that knowledge was almost lost, but the last couple of decades have seen a renewed interest in herbal remedies, and more and more people are recognizing the many benefits of using them to treat themselves and their family.

Used appropriately, herbs can be a satisfying part of a more holistic lifestyle, and many herbs are of course the starting point of much of the modern medicine used today. When used with common sense, herbal remedies are a safe and effective form of home help. If we can treat colds, flu, or minor injuries in the early stages we can often prevent the development of something more serious and avoid using conventional drugs with their risk of side-effects.

Learning which herbs work for us enables us to learn more about the plants that surround us, as well as our own healing processes. However, some herbs are not suitable for everyone or at every stage of life (during pregnancy, for example); if in any doubt you should always consult a medical practitioner.

We have "tried and tested" all the recipes in this book, so we can promise they are delicious as well as being good for you. We are excited to have the opportunity to introduce you to some more unusual plants and flavours so you can be more adventurous whilst trusting that your health and well-being will benefit.

Neal's Yard Remedies has over thirty years of expertise and passion in creating wonderful, natural hair- and skincare products and we are delighted to share some of our favourite ways of using herbs to heal and nurture your skin. Enjoy creating and using your own herbal remedies!

Susan Curtis, Natural Health Director, Neal's Yard Remedies

Consultant's note

Hippocrates, the father of medicine, wrote: "Let food be thy medicine, and medicine be thy food". Many herbs described in this book are used both as tasty foods and as medicines, and the delicious recipes provide new ideas for combining healthy ingredients. Although the herbal medicines have not yet all been researched by modern science, most have stood the test of time. You should always see your doctor for serious health problems, but I hope this book will help readers to treat and prevent minor illnesses, and to understand treatments prescribed by their herbalist.

Dr Merlin Willcox MRCGP MCPP

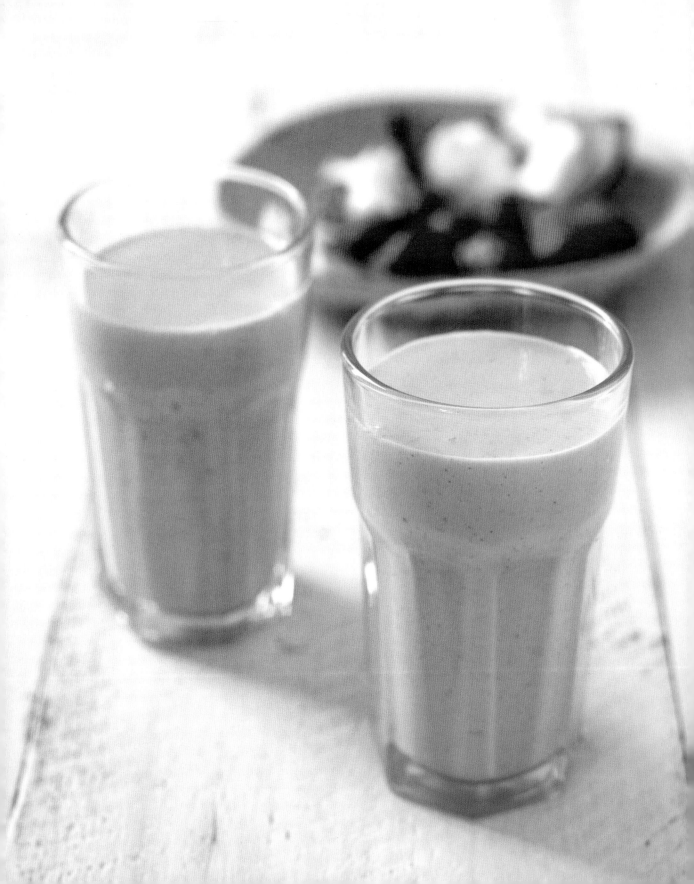

MAKING JUICES AND SMOOTHIES

These juice recipes provide an instant means of detoxing and revitalizing your body, while the smoothies are a healthy yet tasty way to combine fruits, seeds, grains, and nuts to provide vitamins, minerals, phytonutrients (from fruit), essential fatty acids, and protein (from seeds).

Strawberry and macadamia smoothie

 ACTS AS A MALE TONIC

INGREDIENTS
½ vanilla pod
50g (1¾oz) raw macadamia nuts
pulp of 1 young medium-sized
  coconut
250g (9oz) fresh strawberries
a little of the coconut juice (optional)

Makes 4 servings

This healthy twist on strawberries and cream uses an exotic version of cream made from coconut pulp and macadamia nuts. Macadamia nut oil is a rich source of monounsaturated fatty acids, which are reputed to lower cholesterol, while coconut pulp helps to clear the effects of summer heat in the body, quenches the thirst, and is a male reproductive tonic.

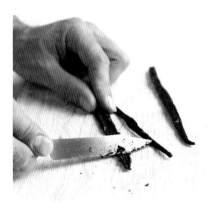

1 Slit the vanilla pod open with a sharp knife, then scrape out the seeds.

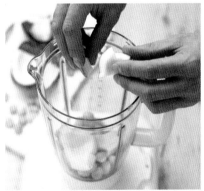

2 Place the nuts and the coconut pulp in a blender or food processor.

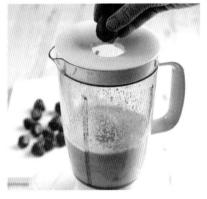

3 Add the strawberries and vanilla seeds. Pulse all the ingredients to give a smooth, silky texture. If the smoothie seems very thick, add enough coconut juice to give it a better texture. Pour into 4 glasses and serve.

Goji berry and pine nut smoothie

 PURIFIES SKIN   **SUPPORTS URINARY SYSTEM**   **SUPPORTS URINARY SYSTEM**

Makes 2 servings

Goji berries provide many amino acids and trace minerals – in particular germanium, a trace mineral thought to have anti-cancer properties. Not surprisingly, they have become known as a "superfruit". The berries are also a rich source of carotenoids, including zeaxanthin (which strengthens eyesight) and vitamins C, B complex, and vitamin E.

INGREDIENTS

50g (1¾oz) almonds
50g (1¾oz) goji berries
  (fresh or dried)
20g (¾oz) pine nuts
1 tsp linseed oil
2–3 leaves of fresh peppermint
350–400ml (12–14fl oz) mineral water
  (start with less water and adjust
  to a consistency and thickness
  you like)

METHOD

1 To sprout the almonds, soak them in cold water for half an hour, then rinse in a colander under running water. Place in a large bowl, cover with water, and leave overnight to soak. The next day, pop the skins off, place the almonds in a clean bowl, pour over mineral water, and refrigerate for up to 24 hours before draining.
2 Wash the goji berries and, if dried, soak them for few hours in a bowl of mineral water (allow enough space for the berries to expand and sufficient water – 150ml/5fl oz of water should be enough – for the fruit to remain submerged). Drain the berries.
3 Place all ingredients in a blender or food processor and blend with the mineral water to give a smooth silky texture. If the consistency is a bit too thick, add a little more water and blend.

Blackcurrant booster smoothie

 RELIEVES INFLAMMATION   **PROTECTS BRAIN**

Makes 2 servings

Blackcurrants are rich in vitamin C, rutin, and other flavonoids. Their high essential fatty acid levels may help to treat inflammatory conditions and manage pain, as well as regulate the circulatory system and enhance the immune system. Use warm rice milk and add a little more roasted barley and some nuts to turn this smoothie into a nourishing breakfast in winter.

INGREDIENTS

50g (1¾oz) fresh blackcurrants
  (or used dried and soak first)
50g (1¾oz) roasted barley
4 tsp agave syrup
4 tsp coconut oil
250ml (9fl oz) rice milk (unsweetened)
A little mineral water

METHOD

Put all the ingredients except the mineral water in a blender or food processor and blend until smooth. Add enough mineral water to ensure the smoothie is of a pourable consistency.

Sour cherry and raw cocoa smoothie

 REGULATES SLEEP

Makes 2 servings

This smoothie is ideal before or after exercising and for long-distance runners, as the anti-inflammatory properties of cherries aid quicker muscle recovery and pain relief. Sour cherries are also a source of natural melatonin, a potent antioxidant with immune system-modulating properties. If eaten regularly, they may even help to regulate the body's natural sleep patterns.

INGREDIENTS
50g (1¾oz) sour cherries, stoned
  if fresh, or dried
300ml (10fl oz) rice or almond milk
4 tsp raw or regular cocoa powder
4 tsp hemp seeds, shelled
4 tsp flaxseed oil

METHOD
1 If using dried sour cherries, soak them for few hours in 150ml (5fl oz) of mineral water.
2 Combine half the rice or almond milk with the rest of the ingredients in a blender or food processor and blend to a smooth, silky, pourable consistency. Add the rest of the milk in stages until the texture of the smoothie is to your liking.

Almond and rose smoothie

 HARMONIZES EMOTIONS **MOISTURIZES SKIN**

Makes 2 servings

Almonds are a great food for strengthening the heart and blood vessels. They contain nutrients such as magnesium, potassium, copper, selenium, manganese, and vitamin E, which is known for its antioxidant activity. Almonds are also reported to lower cholesterol levels, while rose creates a sense of relaxed well-being.

INGREDIENTS
50g (1¾oz) almonds
300–400ml (10–14fl oz) mineral water
2½ tbsp rose syrup
4 tsp almond oil
1 drop rose attar essential oil
  (optional)
8 damask rose petals (optional)

METHOD
1 To sprout the almonds, soak them in cold water for half an hour, then rinse in a colander under running water. Place in a large bowl, cover with water, and leave overnight to soak. The next day, pop the skins off, place the almonds in a clean bowl, pour over filtered or bottled mineral water, and refrigerate for up to 24 hours before draining. Discard the soaking water.
2 Combine half the mineral water with the rest of the ingredients in a blender or food processor and blend to a smooth, silky, pourable consistency. Add the rest of the water in stages until the texture of the smoothie is to your liking.

Garden greens juice

 DETOXES

Makes 2 servings

If you have a vegetable garden, a great way to use up any excess produce is to serve it as refreshing, detoxifying drinks. Courgettes, cucumber, and celery stems all provide a mild base to which you can add fragrant cabbage leaves, sour chard, and spinach. The marjoram added to this juice aids digestion and alleviates abdominal distension and wind.

INGREDIENTS

2 handfuls of kale leaves
2 Swiss chard leaves
1 large handful of spinach leaves
½ cucumber
1 small green courgette
3 stems celery
2 dandelion leaves (large)
2 stems fresh marjoram
a dash of lemon juice (optional)

METHOD

Wash and juice all the vegetables and herbs, and mix thoroughly. Add the lemon juice to taste if you wish or, if you prefer a more powerful lemon flavour, add an eighth of a lemon (organic is preferable) and mix well until blended.

Red pepper and sprouted seeds juice

 STIMULATES DIGESTION   **STIMULATES CIRCULATION**

Makes 2 servings

This fragrant, spicy juice is a great way to start the day. Chilli stimulates the body, particularly the circulation, strengthens the digestive system, and provides a sense of vigour and warmth, which is beneficial in winter. It also causes the body to perspire, and therefore cool down, which can help during periods of hot weather.

INGREDIENTS

1 red pepper, deseeded and
   cut into quarters
20g (¾oz) sprouted alfalfa seeds
20g (¾oz) sprouted red clover seeds
10g (¼oz) sprouted broccoli seeds
½ cucumber
2–3 fresh mint leaves
½ small fresh red chilli, deseeded

METHOD

Juice all the ingredients and mix thoroughly.

Ginger and fennel juice

 SOOTHES INFLAMED
SKIN
 IMPROVES DIGESTION

Makes 2 servings

Fennel bulb, celery, cucumber, and courgette have a cooling, anti-inflammatory effect on the body, and are beneficial for inflammatory conditions in the stomach, lungs, throat, skin, and vagina. They are also diuretic, as well as purifying the skin and moistening the lungs. Ginger and basil are included to add fragrance, remove any bloated feelings, and improve digestion.

INGREDIENTS
1 large fennel bulb
1cm (½in) cube fresh ginger
  root, peeled
2 celery stems
½ small cucumber
½ small green courgette
1 stem fresh basil

METHOD
Juice all the ingredients, mix well, and drink immediately.

Fennel and broccoli sprouts juice

 RESTORES PH BALANCE
 IMPROVES DIGESTION

Makes 2 servings

This juice aims to expel body waste by increasing urination and clearing the bowels to eliminate putrefactive bacteria. Broccoli sprouts are also beneficial for inflammatory eye conditions, while carrots, fennel, and alfalfa seeds are alkaline-forming and help to clear acidic conditions, thus helping rheumatism.

INGREDIENTS
1 large fennel bulb
45g (1½oz) sprouted broccoli seeds
45g (1½oz) sprouted alfalfa seeds
1 large carrot
2 stems celery
2–3 fresh mint leaves
dash of lemon juice

METHOD
Juice all the ingredients, add the lemon juice to taste, and mix well.

Early autumn rambler's delight

 ENHANCES RESISTANCE TO COLDS AND FLU

Makes 2 servings

This is a great way to use freshly picked elderberries and blackberries, which contain high levels of antioxidants that help to fight free-radical damage and enhance the immune system. Blackberries are extremely high in phenolic compounds, which are known to be health-promoting, antiviral, and antibacterial, while elderberries contain potassium and vitamins C and E.

INGREDIENTS

3½ apples, peeled, cored, and chopped
⅓ pear peeled, cored, and chopped
12 ripe elderberries, rinsed, with all stalks removed
20 ripe blackberries, rinsed

METHOD

1 Put all the ingredients into a blender or a food processor and blend until smooth.
2 Divide between two glasses and top with elderberry and elderflower cordial to enhance the antiviral content of the smoothie.

NOTE: Unripe raw elderberries and elder bark should be avoided, so make sure you use completely ripe elderberries with no stalk attached to make this smoothie.

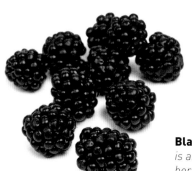

Blackberry (*Rubus fruticosus*)
is an astringent, tonic, mildly diuretic herb, often to be found growing wild in hedgerows.

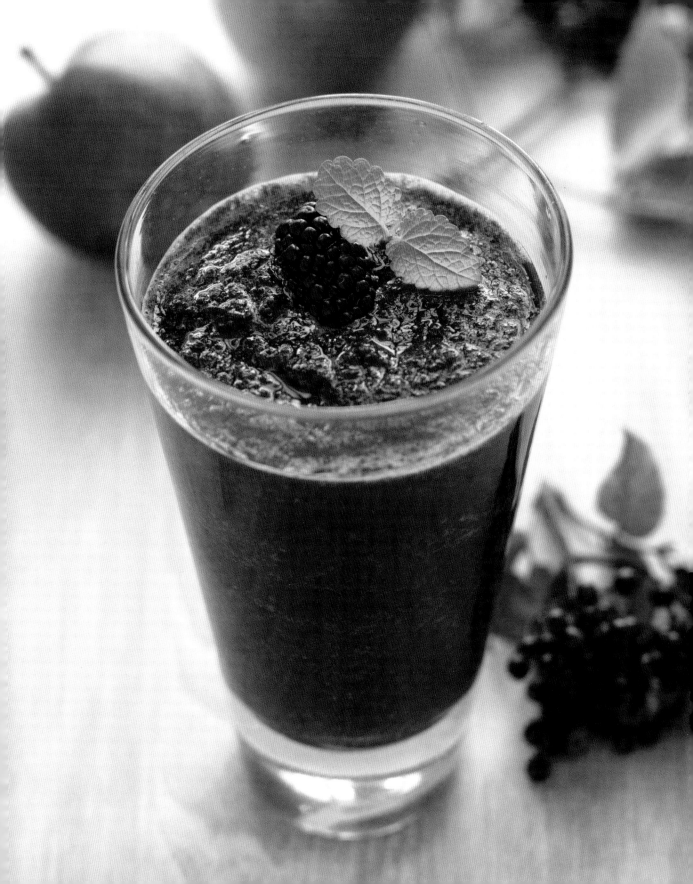

Buckwheat greens and pea shoot juice

 STRENGTHENS BLOOD VESSELS

Makes 2 servings

Pea shoots and buckwheat greens are excellent sources of enzymes, vitamins, and chlorophyll. Buckwheat also contains rutin (4–6 per cent), which strengthens the capillaries (rutin belongs to a group of plant compounds called bioflavonoids – powerful antioxidants that fight free radicals) and is useful for reducing varicose veins and haemorrhoids.

INGREDIENTS

2 tbsp young buckwheat greens, finely chopped
4 tbsp fresh pea shoots
2 courgettes
1 cucumber
2 tbsp fresh marjoram leaves
a dash of lemon juice
200ml (7fl oz) mineral water

METHOD

Juice all ingredients, add the mineral water and lemon juice to taste, and mix well.

Tomato salsa juice

 IMPROVES DIGESTION   **ENHANCES WELL-BEING AND CONFIDENCE**

Makes 2 servings

This is a great juice to make when you feel like something substantial and savoury, but have no time to make a cooked meal. Basil has a reputation for restoring the vital spirits, quickening the brain, and awakening joy and courage. It also enhances digestion, clears respiratory congestion and phlegm, and lifts depression.

INGREDIENTS

5 ripe tomatoes
½ cucumber
1 small clove of garlic
½ fresh red chilli, deseeded
1 stem fresh basil leaves
2 stems celery
1 tsp virgin olive oil
salt to taste
1 red pepper, deseeded

METHOD

Juice all the vegetables and herbs, add the olive oil, season to taste with a little salt if you wish, and mix well. If you prefer your juice red, add 1 deseeded red pepper to the vegetables and herbs when you juice them.

Artichoke leaf and fennel juice

 DETOXES   **COMBATS NEGATIVE EMOTIONS**

Makes 2 servings

The liver needs help every now and then to eliminate wastes from the body. Artichoke leaves, which have a strong, bitter taste, contain cynarin, a compound that stimulates the liver to release these toxic substances and which also improves liver function. Fennel, dandelion leaves, celery stems, and courgette also enhance the elimination of waste through the kidneys.

INGREDIENTS

1 tsp artichoke leaves (from a globe artichoke plant), finely chopped
1 medium fennel bulb
4 fresh dandelion leaves
4 celery stems
½ courgette

METHOD

Juice all the ingredients, mix thoroughly, and drink. If you find the juice overly bitter, dilute it with some mineral water until it tastes palatable.

Sunflower greens and wheatgrass juice

 DETOXES   **REJUVENATES, REVITALIZES**

Makes 2 servings

The juice from wheatgrass and sunflower greens (young plants) is a natural aid that can be used in the treatment of degenerative diseases and to help slow cellular deterioration and relieve inflammation. Its high chlorophyll content also helps to detoxify the liver, so cleansing and energizing the body.

INGREDIENTS

100g (3½oz) sunflower greens
100g (3½oz) wheatgrass blades
300ml (10fl oz) or more mineral water to dilute to taste

METHOD

Juice the sunflower greens and wheatgrass, blend well, and add enough mineral water to dilute the flavour of the juice and give it a palatable taste.

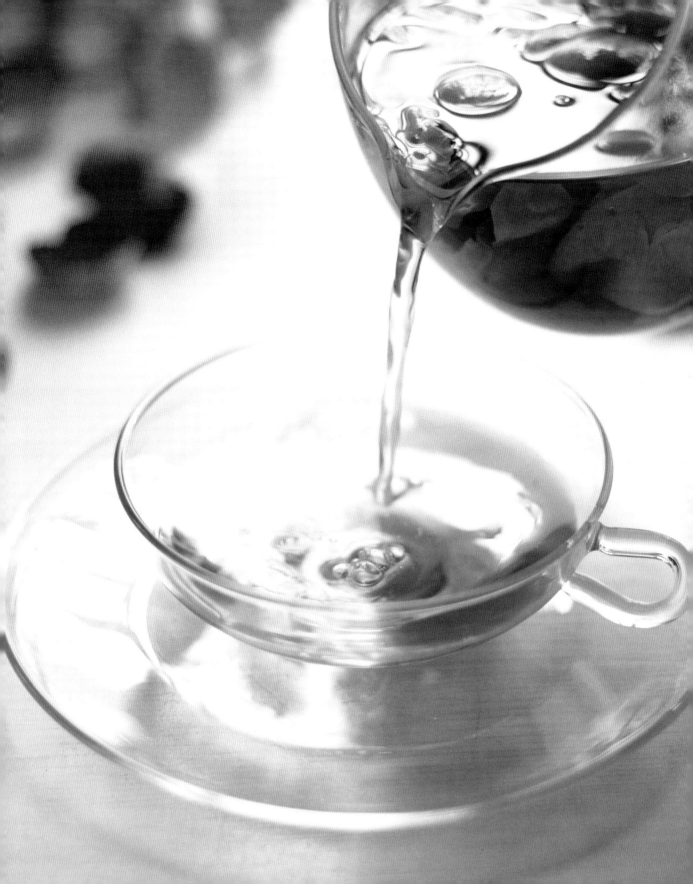

MAKING TEAS

The recipes for the tea blends provided here allow you to explore the wonderful flavours of plants, with subtle nurturing and healing qualities in a single cup. All the plants mentioned here can be used either fresh or dry – and may inspire you to grow your own healing teas in your garden.

Lemon balm and rose tea

 ENHANCES MOOD

Makes 2–3 servings

This herbal tea contains a fusion of empowering yet relaxing lemon balm and mood-enhancing, sensual rose petals to make the ultimate summer refreshment. It can be enjoyed hot or cold, and is best drunk slightly bitter. For the best results, pick fresh lemon balm leaves and fresh perfumed rose petals from the damask rose (*Rosa* x *damascena*) or French rose (*Rosa gallica*).

INGREDIENTS

16 leaves of fresh lemon balm (the soft flowering tops can also be used), or 1 tbsp dried lemon balm

2 rose heads with petals removed, or 2 tbsp dried rose petals

METHOD

1 Put the fresh lemon balm leaves and rose petals in a large teapot. If using dried lemon balm and rose petals, spoon them into the teapot instead.

2 Boil 500ml (16fl oz) of water, allow to cool for 5 minutes, then pour it into the teapot. Allow to infuse for 5 minutes and then serve. More water can be added later if needed to re-infuse the leaves and rose petals.

Chamomile and fennel tea

 IMPROVES DIGESTION

Makes 3 servings

This is a soothing, anti-inflammatory infusion of herbs that are well known for their beneficial effect on an unsettled, bloated or acidic digestive system. It will encourage better food assimilation, help to regulate the bowels and improve an over-acidic system.

INGREDIENTS

1 tsp chamomile flowers

1 tsp fennel seeds

1 tsp meadowsweet

1 tsp marshmallow root, finely chopped

1 tsp yarrow

METHOD

1 Put the herbs in a large teapot.

2 Boil 500ml (16fl oz) of boiling water, and add to the teapot. Allow to infuse for 5 minutes and serve. Drink 1 mug of the infusion 2–3 times a day.

NOTE: This tea is not suitable for use during pregnancy.

Dandelion and burdock tea

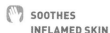 SOOTHES
INFLAMED SKIN

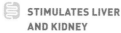 STIMULATES LIVER
AND KIDNEY

Makes 3–4 servings

This classic blend of herbs helps to clear up blemished skin. It treats eczema and acne by gently invigorating the liver and kidneys to remove accumulated waste, while its anti-inflammatory activity helps to improve skin eruptions on the head, neck, and upper body.

INGREDIENTS
1 tsp dandelion leaves
1 tsp burdock leaves
1 tsp cleavers herb
1 tsp red clover flowers

METHOD
Place all the ingredients in a teapot, pour in 500ml (16fl oz) of boiling water, allow to infuse for 10–15 minutes, and serve. Drink hot or cold through the day.

NOTE: This tea is not suitable for use during pregnancy.

Yarrow and calendula tea

 RELIEVES PMS

 HARMONIZES EMOTIONS

 IMPROVES
CIRCULATION

Makes 3–4 servings

These herbs all benefit the female body. Yarrow and calendula relieve blood and energy stagnation in the abdomen and improve blood circulation to the womb. Vervain invigorates the liver, releases tension, and relaxes the mind. Lady's mantle, an astringent, relieves congestion through urination. Raspberry leaf will help to relieve period pains.

INGREDIENTS
1 tsp yarrow
1 tsp marigold flowers
1 tsp lady's mantle
1 tsp vervain
1 tsp raspberry leaf

METHOD
Place all the ingredients in a teapot, pour in 500ml (16fl oz) of boiling water, allow to infuse for 10–15 minutes, and serve. Drink hot or cold through the day. Take 2–4 cups with the onset of pain, and reassess with your health professional if the pain persists.

NOTE: This tea is not suitable for use during pregnancy.

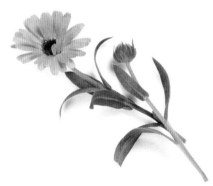

Calendula (Calendula officinalis)
has astringent and anti-inflammatory properties, and the flowers are rich in antioxidants.

Skullcap and orange flower tea

 RELIEVES DEPRESSION

Makes 3–4 servings

Herbal teas such as this can help you to relax and begin to put things into perspective – especially if you are suffering from feelings of depression. Skullcap, St John's wort, wood betony, lemon balm, and orange flower are all known to help to ease tensions, relax the body and mind, and lift the spirits.

INGREDIENTS
1 tsp skullcap
1 tsp orange flowers
1 tsp St. John's wort
1 tsp wood betony
1 tsp lemon balm

METHOD
Place all the ingredients in a teapot, pour in 500ml (16fl oz) of boiling water, allow to infuse for 10–15 minutes, and serve. Drink hot or cold through the day.

NOTE: This tea is not suitable for use during pregnancy.

Blackberry and wild strawberry tea

 DETOXES

Makes 3–4 servings

The leaves of these fruits are well known for their ability to heal, as well as for their revitalizing and rejuvenating qualities. Their ability to cleanse the body of the excesses of winter is remarkable. Use fresh leaves to make this tea in the spring, and harvest and dry some for use during the winter months.

INGREDIENTS
2 tsp blackberry leaves
1 tsp wild strawberry leaves
1 tsp raspberry leaves
1 tsp blackcurrant leaves

METHOD
Place all the ingredients in a teapot, pour in 500ml (16fl oz) of boiling water, allow to infuse for 10–15 minutes, and serve. Drink hot or cold through the day.

NOTE: This tea is not suitable for use during pregnancy.

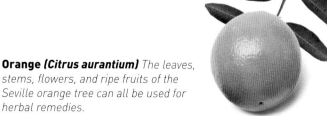

Orange (Citrus aurantium) *The leaves, stems, flowers, and ripe fruits of the Seville orange tree can all be used for herbal remedies.*

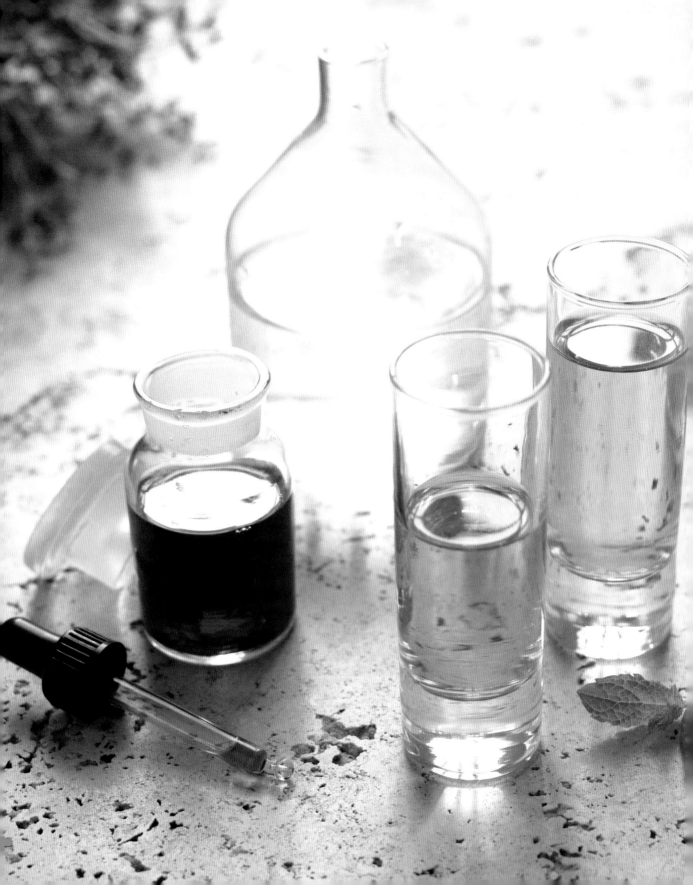

HOW TO MAKE TINCTURES

Tinctures are concentrated, alcohol-based extracts of plant materials, and are much more portable and long-lasting than herbal teas. These recipes enable you to produce simple extracts and further explore the benefits of medicinal herbs.

Peppermint and thyme tincture

 CALMS A NERVOUS GUT

INGREDIENTS
25g (scant 1oz) peppermint
15g (½oz) thyme
25g (scant 1oz) chamomile
20g (¾oz) yarrow
15g (½oz) liquorice root
500ml (16fl oz) good-quality vodka

Makes approx 500ml (16fl oz)

This tincture tastes good enough to serve as an aperitif. It aids digestion and benefits the activity of the large intestine, and helps to expel wind and soothe a nervous stomach. Use within 6 months.

NOTE: This tincture is not suitable for use during pregnancy.

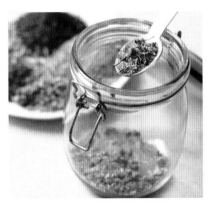

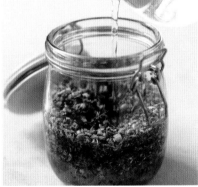

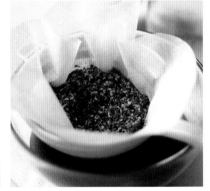

1 *Place all the ingredients* except the vodka in a large jar.

2 *Cover with the vodka,* stir, and make sure all the ingredients are well immersed. Seal the jar tightly and place it in a dark cupboard. Give the jar a few good shakes every day for 3 weeks.

3 *Open the jar* and strain the ingredients through a muslin-lined sieve into a shallow bowl. Discard the ingredients in the muslin and pour the liquid into an amber glass bottle. Label the tincture bottle with the names of all the ingredients and the date. Take 1 teaspoon in a glass of warm or cold water and sip before or after meals.

Dandelion and burdock tincture

 DETOXES

Makes 300–350ml (10–12fl oz)

The toxic environment many of us now live in puts enormous strain on the liver, so good liver health is more important than ever before. This tincture of bitter herbs stimulates the liver to metabolize toxic residues, and influences the rest of the digestive system. It also improves the blood circulation and helps to make you feel calmer and less irritable.

INGREDIENTS

20g (¾oz) dandelion root
20g (¾oz) burdock root
20g (¾oz) schisandra berries
10g (¼oz) artichoke leaves
20g (¾oz) milk thistle
10g (¼oz) gentian root
  (*Gentiana lutea*)
400ml (14fl oz) good-quality vodka

METHOD

1 Ensure that all the dried ingredients are finely chopped, but not powdered.
2 Place all the ingredients except the vodka into a large glass jar with a secure-fitting lid. Pour in the vodka, close the lid tightly, and shake a few times.
3 Label the jar with all the ingredients and the date. Place the jar in a dark cupboard and shake it at least once every day for 3 weeks.
4 Strain the contents of the jar through a muslin bag into a measuring jug and pour the tincture into an appropriately sized (350–400ml/12–14fl oz) sterilized amber glass bottle. Seal the bottle.
5 Label with all the ingredients and the original starting date. Start by taking a few drops each day and build up to 1 teaspoon 2–3 times a day. Use within 6 months.

NOTE: This tincture is not suitable for use during pregnancy.

Crampbark and valerian tincture

🔲 **RELIEVES MINOR PAIN**   🔘 **RELIEVES PERIOD PAINS**

Makes 300–350ml (10–12fl oz)

This blend relieves broad-spectrum spasmodic pain due to stress, including discomfort associated with irritability, disturbed sleep, and nervous indigestion. Crampbark helps relieve smooth muscle spasms, valerian and passionflower provide a mild sedative effect and relieve irritability, and chamomile has an anti-inflammatory and antispasmodic effect.

INGREDIENTS
25g (scant 1oz) crampbark
25g (scant 1oz) valerian root
20g (¾oz) passionflower
20g (¾oz) chamomile
400ml (14fl oz) good-quality vodka

METHOD

1 Ensure that all the dried ingredients are finely chopped, but not powdered.

2 Place all the ingredients except the vodka into a large glass jar with a secure-fitting lid. Pour in the vodka, close the lid tightly, and shake a few times.

3 Label the jar with all the ingredients and the date. Place the jar in a dark cupboard and shake it at least once every day for 3 weeks.

4 Strain the contents of the jar through a muslin bag into a measuring jug and pour the tincture into an appropriately sized (350–400ml/12–14fl oz) sterilized amber glass bottle. Seal the bottle.

5 Label with all the ingredients and the original starting date. Start by taking a few drops each day and build up to 1 teaspoon 2–3 times a day. Use within 6 months.

NOTE: This tincture is not suitable for use during pregnancy.

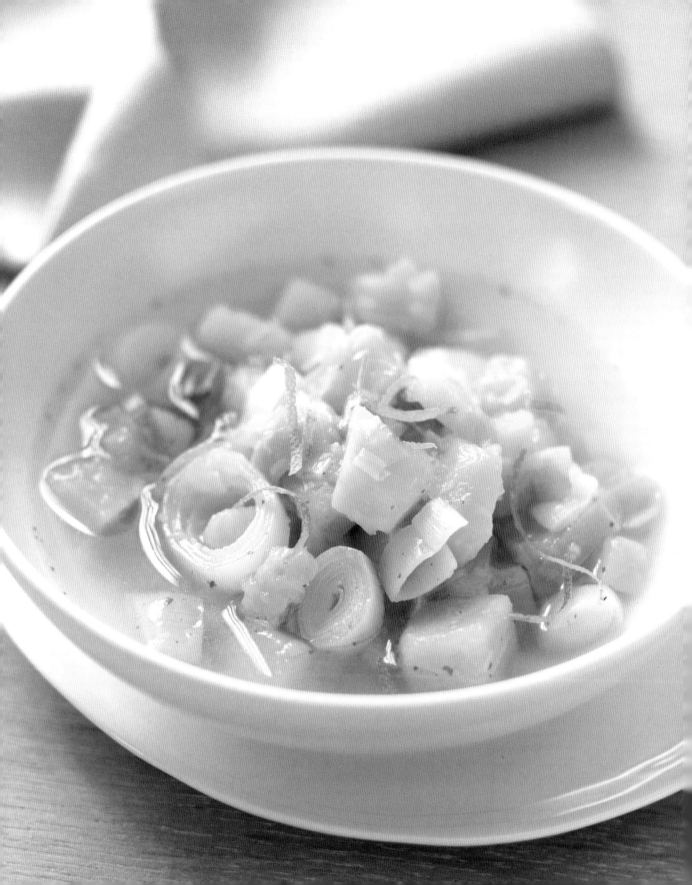

MAKING SOUPS

Soups have a history of being used as a healing aid, especially for anyone recovering from an illness. These recipes have been specially devised to include essential, life-generating plant ingredients; they all taste delicious as well as doing you good.

Onion squash and ginger soup

 WARMS AND NOURISHES

Makes 4–6 servings

This is a great warming winter soup with a hint of the Orient. Ginger is famous for its healing qualities, and fresh ginger is traditionally used to ward off winter ailments: it acts as a diaphoretic, warms up the body, and helps in the elimination of cold. It also improves the digestion and assimilation of nutrients.

INGREDIENTS

2 tbsp olive oil
1kg (2¼lb) onion squash (or butternut squash), peeled, deseeded, and cut into small chunks
1 medium-sized leek, sliced
4 cloves of garlic, crushed
2 tbsp fresh ginger root, grated
1.5 litres (2¾ pints) vegetable stock
lime juice and zest to taste
salt and freshly ground black pepper

METHOD

1 Heat the olive oil in a saucepan, add the squash and leek, and sauté for few minutes. Add the garlic and ginger and a splash of the stock and continue to sauté the ingredients until the leek is soft. Add rest of the stock and bring to the boil. Simmer for approximately 10 minutes or until the squash is cooked through, but still retains some shape.
2 Remove from the heat, add the lime juice and a sprinkle of the lime zest, and season to taste. The soup can be served as it is, or blended until smooth.

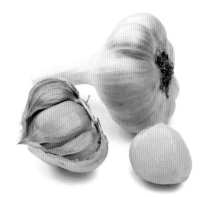

Garlic (Allium sativum)
Garlic is a popular culinary herb that can ward off bacterial infection. It keeps its flavour well when cooked.

Green bean and coriander soup

 CLEANSES

Makes 4 servings

This soup helps to balance blood-sugar levels: research has shown that bean pods contain a substance (arginine) that acts like insulin by regulating blood-sugar levels in the body, although it is weaker and acts more slowly over a prolonged period of time. Bean pods are also known to have a diuretic affect.

INGREDIENTS

2 large potatoes, peeled and diced
2 tbsp olive oil
1 onion, finely chopped
2 carrots, scrubbed and finely sliced
1kg (2¼lb) green beans (preferably yellow), topped, tailed, and sliced
3 garlic cloves, chopped
1 chilli pepper, deseeded and finely chopped
1–2 tsp picante pimenton (hot smoked paprika)
salt and freshly ground black pepper to taste
4 tbsp fresh coriander leaves, finely chopped
4 tbsp half-fat crème fraiche to serve (1 tbsp per serving)

METHOD

1 Place the potatoes in a pot, cover with water, and bring to the boil.
2 In the meantime, warm the oil in a frying pan, add the onion, and sauté until soft. Add the carrots to the frying pan, stir, and continue to sauté for few minutes. Add the beans, stir, cover the pan, turn the heat down low, and allow to sweat. Then add the chopped garlic, chilli pepper, and the smoked paprika.
3 Check that the vegetables are giving off enough juices to prevent the bottom of the pan burning; if necessary add a spoonful or two of water (the idea is that the vegetables cook in their own juices).
4 When the beans are nearly ready (soft, but chewy), add the cooked potatoes to the frying pan and add just a small amount of the water in which the potatoes were cooked.
5 Cook all the vegetables together for a few more minutes so that they combine well. Season to taste.
6 Serve the soup in bowls garnished with fresh coriander leaves and a spoonful of crème fraiche.

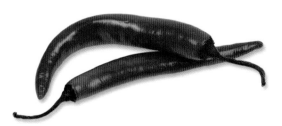

Chilli/cayenne pepper (Capsicum frutescens) *Warming red chillies and dried cayenne pepper stimulate circulation and aid digestion.*

Burdock root and carrot soup

 CLEANSING

Makes 4 servings

This is a gentle, cleansing soup for the body. Burdock root is often used in the treatment of skin conditions and eczema, as well as rheumatic complaints, and is also famous as a blood purifier. It is grown commercially as a root vegetable and can be found most readily in Asian, especially Japanese, greengrocers.

INGREDIENTS

3 shallots, finely chopped
100g (3½oz) fresh burdock root, washed and finely chopped
3 large carrots, washed and finely chopped
2 small garlic cloves, finely chopped
salt and freshly ground black pepper
1 tbsp fresh lovage leaves, finely shredded, to garnish
a drizzle of pumpkin seed oil

METHOD

1 Place 2 tablespoons of water into a saucepan, add the shallots, and sauté for 1–2 minutes, stirring occasionally. When the shallots are soft, stir in the burdock root and carrots, keeping the pot covered and the heat turned down low so the vegetables steam in their own juices.
2 Check and stir the ingredients every few minutes and, if necessary, add a little more water. When they are sufficiently soft, add the garlic and cook for another minute. Add 500ml (16fl oz) of boiling water and simmer for 5 minutes.
3 Pour the soup into a blender or food processor and blend until smooth and silky. Season with salt and pepper to taste and serve in individual bowls. Garnish each with shredded lovage leaves and a little pumpkin seed oil.

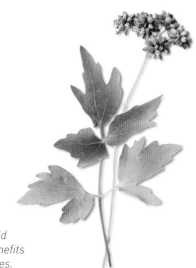

Lovage (Levisticum officinale)
Lovage contains quercetin, a flavonoid reputed to have numerous health benefits including anti-inflammatory properties.

Nettle and sweet potato soup

 PURIFIES SKIN   **ACTS AS A SPRINGTIME TONIC**

Makes 4 servings

Nettle soup has been used as a health tonic for generations in Europe; nettles are full of vitamins and minerals and purify the blood, clear toxins, lower blood pressure, and improve skin and hair.

INGREDIENTS

1 tbsp olive oil
1 medium-sized onion, or
  4 shallots, chopped
1 medium-sized sweet potato,
  chopped into small pieces
2 garlic cloves, squeezed
1 litre (1¾ pints) vegetable stock
250g (9oz) young nettle leaves,
  washed and chopped
salt and freshly ground black pepper
2–3 tbsp barley miso paste
4 tsp half-fat crème fraîche, or
  plain yoghurt

METHOD

1 Heat the oil in a saucepan and sauté the onions or shallots and sweet potato for 2–3 minutes. Add the garlic and stock and bring to the boil. Simmer for 20 minutes, then add the nettles and turn off the heat.

2 Pour the soup into a blender or food processor and blend until smooth.

3 Season to taste with salt and pepper and the miso paste. Serve in individual bowls, each with a swirl (1 teaspoon) of crème fraiche or yoghurt.

Courgette and sea greens soup

 ASSISTS WEIGHT CONTROL   **ASSISTS WEIGHT CONTROL**

Makes 4 servings

Seaweed is also known for its ability to help remove toxic waste from the body, improve kidney function, alkalize the blood, assist in weight control, and lower cholesterol.

INGREDIENTS

1 handful dried wakame seaweed,
  or any other colourful soft-leaf
  seaweed such as dulse
4 shallots, chopped
1 medium-sized fennel bulb, chopped
5 medium-sized courgettes, sliced
1 tbsp fresh parsley, finely chopped
salt and freshly ground black pepper
  to taste
a drizzle of pumpkin seed oil

METHOD

1 Soak the seaweed in at least 600ml (1 pint) of clean water.

2 Place a tablespoon of water in a saucepan and heat. Add the chopped shallots and cook over a low heat with the lid on, stirring occasionally.

3 When soft, add the fennel and courgettes. Continue to cook the vegetables with the lid on until they are tender.

4 Drain the seaweed. Place the cooked vegetables in a blender or food processor, add the chopped parsley and 500–600ml (16fl oz–1 pint) of water, and blend until smooth. Add salt and black pepper to taste.

5 Divide the rehydrated seaweed leaves into 4 piles, pour the soup into individual bowls, and scatter the seaweed over the top of each serving. Sprinkle over the fresh parlsey and a little of the pumpkin seed oil and serve.

Ginseng and astragalus longevity soup

 ENERGIZING   **ENHANCES DIGESTION**

Makes 4 servings

The energizing ingredients in this soup include ginseng, which enhances energy levels and restores strength after a prolonged illness, and astragalus root, which is well known for its beneficial effect on the immune system. It strengthens the lungs, helps to prevent colds, and alleviates any shortness of breath. Chinese black fungus is rich in amino acids, phosphorus, iron, and calcium.

INGREDIENTS

15g (½oz) Chinese black fungus (hei mu er/*Auricularia auricula*)
15g (½oz) fresh or dried astragalus root
15g (½oz) fresh or dried ginseng root
6 shallots, topped and tailed with the skins left on
3 garlic cloves, topped and tailed with the skins left on
1 large carrot, scrubbed
2.5cm (1in) cube fresh ginger root, thinly sliced
150g (5½oz) fresh shiitake mushrooms
150g (5½oz) fresh oyster mushrooms
1 large piece wakame seaweed, cut into small pieces, or 1 tbsp dried
15g (½oz) goji berries, pre-soaked if dried
200g (7oz) buckwheat or soba, noodles
2–3 tbsp barley miso paste
1 handful of flat-leaf parsley, chopped
freshly ground black pepper

METHOD

1 Put the fungus, astragalus root, ginseng root, shallots, garlic, whole carrot, and ginger into a large saucepan, cover with 1.5 litres (2¾ pints) of water and bring to the boil. Simmer on a very low heat for half an hour with the lid on tightly.

2 Take the pan off the heat, strain the liquid through a colander or sieve, and return it to the pan. Discard the astragalus root and ginseng. Squeeze the garlic and shallots from their skins and return them to the soup. Slice the fungus and carrot into small pieces and return them to the soup. Add the mushrooms and wakame seaweed and bring the soup back to simmering point. Add the goji berries. After 10 minutes, add the buckwheat noodles and let them cook through for 5–7 minutes.

3 Serve in individual bowls. Allow each person to add enough barley miso paste to their liking and garnish with the parsley and a grinding of black pepper.

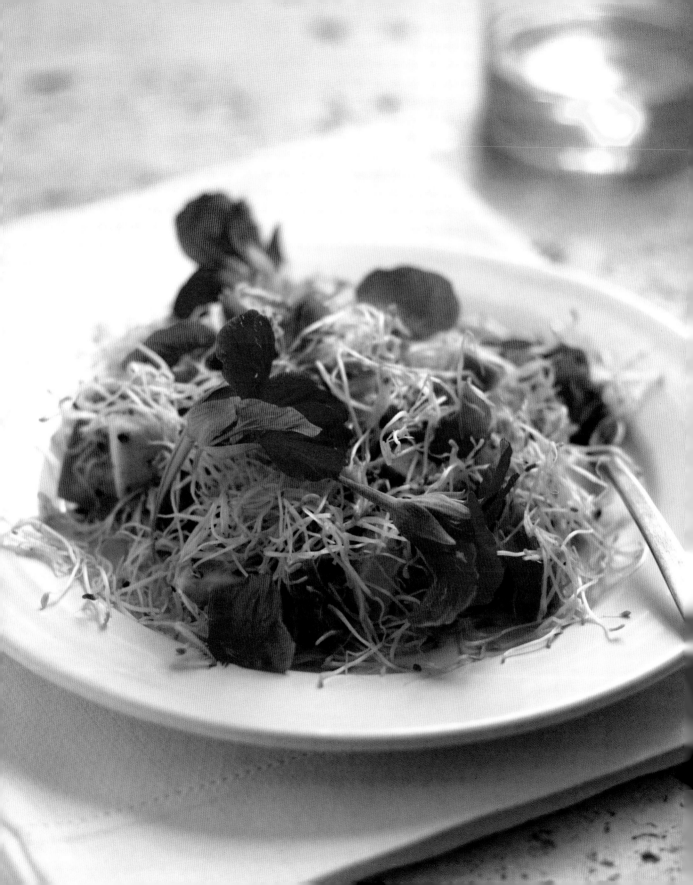

MAKING SALADS

Raw vegetables and herbs are the essence of nourishment, providing nutrients, fluids, and fibre and enhancing the elimination of wastes. These salads combine the healing qualities of fresh vegetables with phytonutrients from herbs, and bring health awareness to the eating experience.

Nasturtium and sprouted seed salad

 DETOXES

Makes 2 servings

Sprouted seeds are a great source of fresh nutrients. Sprouts in general are a mineral-rich food; they often have diuretic and bowel-regulating properties, and are therefore important foods in a detox regime. Nasturtiums flowers impart a delicately peppery taste to this salad. As a medicine, they are thought to have a beneficial influence on the lungs and kidneys.

INGREDIENTS
75g (2½oz) alfalfa sprouts
1 avocado, chopped
1 large tomato, chopped
8 nasturtium flowers

FOR THE DRESSING
1 tbsp olive oil
juice of ½ lemon
¼ tsp mustard
salt and freshly ground black
   pepper, to taste

METHOD
1 Rinse the alfalfa sprouts thoroughly in a colander under running water, then dry them well in a salad spinner or with a clean tea cloth.
2 Mix all the dressing ingredients together and blend well to create a smooth vinaigrette.
3 Place the alfalfa sprouts in a serving bowl and add the avocado and tomato. Pour over the dressing and mix thoroughly. Top the salad with the nasturtium flowers, and serve.

Sauerkraut and avocado salad

REPLENISHES GUT FLORA

Makes 2 servings

Fermented foods such as sauerkraut play an important role in enhancing intestinal health by promoting the growth of organisms that increase nutrient absorption. Cabbage also contains compounds that support colon and breast health, and has antioxidant, antibacterial, and antiviral properties. Once prepared, sauerkraut actually contains more vitamin C than fresh cabbage.

FOR THE SAUERKRAUT
2 medium white cabbages
2 tbsp salt

FOR THE SALAD
50g (1¾oz) alfalfa sprouts, washed
1 avocado, stoned, peeled, and sliced
1 tbsp pumpkin oil
freshly ground black pepper to taste

METHOD

1 To make the sauerkraut (fermented cabbage), shred the cabbage finely in a food processor, pack into a bowl, sprinkle with salt, mix thoroughly, and leave for half an hour.
2 Pound the cabbage with the end of a rolling pin until the juices start flowing. Fill a sterilized glass jar with the salted cabbage, adding a handful at the time and pounding it down in the jar with the end of a rolling pin each time so that no air is left between the added layers ("beating in" is essential to the success of this process). Firmly compress the layers of cabbage, leaving some space at the top of the jar for the cabbage to expand (the juices may also overflow).
3 Place the jar on a plate, cover with a saucer as wide as the neck of the jar, and store in a well-ventilated cool, but not cold, place (see note below). Check the jar and remove any scum from the top regularly. After 1 week the cabbage will have fermented sufficiently to be eaten, and should keep for at least 2 weeks if refrigerated.
4 To make the salad, combine 125g (4½oz) of the sauerkraut with the rest of the ingredients in a salad bowl and season to taste.

NOTE: You can also buy ready-made sauerkraut, but it is often sterilized and your homemade version will taste much better. The ideal temperature for fermentation is 20–22°C (68–72°F). Fermentation will stop and the cabbage will spoil above 24°C (76°F) or below 13°C (55°F). If your sauerkraut develops a pinkish hue on its surface, goes dark, or is very soft and mushy, it has not fermented properly and should not be eaten.

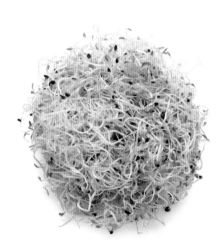

Alfalfa (Medicago sativa) *A flowering plant of the pea family, alfalfa was originally cultivated in the Middle East and is now grown throughout the world.*

Nori rolls

 DETOXES

Makes 3–4 servings

Sheets of nutritious toasted nori seaweed are delicious as part of a healthy snack, and are ideal to use as a wrap filled with fresh vegetables. These rolls make an excellent light, detoxing meal to eat on the go – a true raw food "sandwich". In this recipe the rolls are served as a salad with a tasty dressing.

INGREDIENTS

2 heaped tbsp sesame seeds
5 square sheets toasted nori seaweed
1 small or ½ a large papaya, peeled, deseeded, and cut into thin strips
1 red pepper, deseeded and cut into thin strips
1 chilli, deseeded and cut into thin strips
10cm (4in) inner white part of a leek, sliced thinly lengthways
1 avocado, stoned, peeled, and cut into thin strips

FOR THE DRESSING

juice of 1 lime
1 clove of garlic, crushed
½ tsp fresh ginger root, finely grated
1 tbsp fresh coriander leaves, finely chopped
1 tsp light barley miso paste
½ tsp lime zest
1 tsp maple syrup
3 tbsp mineral water

METHOD

1 Firstly, toast the sesame seeds in a small pan over a low heat for 3–4 minutes, stirring frequently, until they turn lightly golden and begin to release a nutty aroma.
2 To make the dressing, put all the dressing ingredients into a blender or food processor with 1 tablespoon of toasted sesame seeds and blend until smooth.
3 Have a small bowl of water ready. Place a sheet of nori on a sushi mat or a square of greaseproof paper a little longer and wider than the sheet of nori.
4 Put a small amount of each ingredient heaped on top of one another in a line 2–3cm (¾–1¼in) from the edge of the bottom of the nori sheet.
5 Drizzle a little of the dressing over the vegetables and scatter over some of the remaining toasted sesame seeds.
6 Lift the bottom edge of the sushi mat (or paper) and roll up the nori with the ingredients inside. To seal the nori roll, wet your fingers in the small bowl of water, dampen the top edge of the nori sheet, and finish rolling the nori. Repeat with the remaining nori sheets, vegetables, and dressing.
7 When ready to serve, slice the nori rolls into three sections, and stand each one upright on a serving plate. Sprinkle each nori roll with toasted sesame seeds, and use any remaining dressing as a dip.

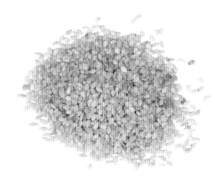

Sesame (Sesamum indicum) *The seeds are exceptionally rich in nutrients and vitamins, including iron, calcium, magnesium, and vitamins B1 and E.*

Gotu kola and ginger body toning cream

 MOISTURIZES SKIN

Makes 40g (1½oz)

This is a nourishing cream with stimulating herbal extracts to restore suppleness and tone. Gotu kola has anti-inflammatory properties and encourages the formation of collagen, which firms and boosts the suppleness of the skin, while ginger, black pepper, and lemon essential oils encourage circulation and help to tone the skin.

INGREDIENTS

1 tbsp apricot oil
2 tbsp gotu kola infusion
2 tsp emulsifying wax
2 drops black pepper essential oil
3 drops ginger essential oil
2 drops lemon essential oil

METHOD

1 Heat the apricot oil in a bowl set over a saucepan of boiling water (bain-marie).
2 Heat the gotu kola infusion and emulsifying wax gently in a saucepan until the emulsifier has dissolved in the infusion.
3 Slowly add the infusion to the apricot oil, stirring constantly. When the mixture has cooled, stir in the essential oils.
4 Store in a sterilized dark glass jar with a tight-fitting lid in the refrigerator, and use within 2 months.

Viola and evening primrose skin cream

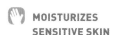 **MOISTURIZES SENSITIVE SKIN**

Makes 40g (1½oz)

A gently soothing and moisturizing skin cream such as this is ideal for sensitive skin. Viola, also known as heartsease, calms and soothes irritated skin and is traditionally used to ease conditions such as eczema. Here it is combined with essential fatty acid-rich avocado and evening primrose oils and gentle chamomile to soothe and nurture delicate skin.

INGREDIENTS

1 tsp lanolin
1 tsp avocado oil
1 tsp evening primrose oil
2 tbsp viola and chamomile infusion (50:50 mix)
10g (¼oz) emulsifying wax

METHOD

1 Melt the lanolin, avocado oil, and evening primrose oil in a bowl set over a saucepan of boiling water (bain-marie).
2 Put the viola and chamomile infusion and emulsifying wax into a saucepan and heat gently until the emulsifier has dissolved.
3 Slowly add the infusion to the lanolin and oil mixture, whisking it together for about 10 seconds.
4 Pour into a sterilized dark glass jar with a tight-fitting lid, store in the refrigerator, and use within 2 months.

Frankincense and wild rose skin cream

 MOISTURIZES SKIN

Makes 40g (1½oz)

Keep skin smooth and radiant with this luxurious facial cream. Frankincense is renowned for its toning, restorative, and anti-ageing properties while rosehip oil helps to improve skin elasticity and prevent moisture loss. Neroli oil, the precious essential oil from the blossom of the bitter orange tree, helps to treat fine lines and encourages a bright, radiant complexion.

INGREDIENTS

½ tsp cocoa butter
1 tsp calendula oil
1 tsp rosehip seed oil
10g (¼oz) emulsifying wax
2 drops frankincense essential oil
1 drop neroli essential oil

METHOD

1 Heat the cocoa butter, calendula oil, and rosehip oil in a bowl set over a saucepan of boiling water (bain-marie).
2 Gently heat the emulsifier and 30ml (2 tbsp) water in a saucepan until the emulsifier has dissolved. Slowly add this to the cocoa butter and oil mixture, whisking it together for about 10 seconds.
3 When the mixture has cooled, stir in the essential oils.
4 Store in a sterilized dark glass jar with a tight-fitting lid in the refrigerator, and use within 2 months.

Cocoa butter and rose body lotion

 MOISTURIZES SKIN

Makes 100ml (3½fl oz)

Antioxidant-rich cocoa butter is deeply nourishing and easily absorbed by the skin. This enriching lotion includes moisturizing, soothing honey and cooling, balancing rose blended with vitamin E rich wheatgerm oil to smooth and soften skin. It has a subtle yet exotic fragrance created by the blend of ylang ylang, benzoin, geranium, and vetiver essential oils.

INGREDIENTS

15g (½oz) cocoa butter
1 tsp lanolin
5 tbsp wheatgerm oil
3 tbsp rose infusion (p.342)
1 tsp honey
25g (scant 1oz) emulsifying wax
5 drops benzoin tincture
5 drops vanilla extract
5 drops ylang ylang essential oil
2 drops rose absolute essential oil
2 drops geranium essential oil
1 drop vetiver essential oil

METHOD

1 Melt the cocoa butter, lanolin, and wheatgerm oil in a bowl set over a pan of boiling water (bain-marie).
2 Make the rose infusion (p.43) and while it is still hot, dissolve the honey and emulsifying wax in it.
3 Add this infusion mixture to the cocoa butter and oil mixture 1 tablespoon at a time, whisking all the while. Then add the benzoin tincture, vanilla extract, and essential oils.
4 Store in a sterilized glass bottle with a tight-fitting lid in the refrigerator for up to 3 weeks. Shake before use.

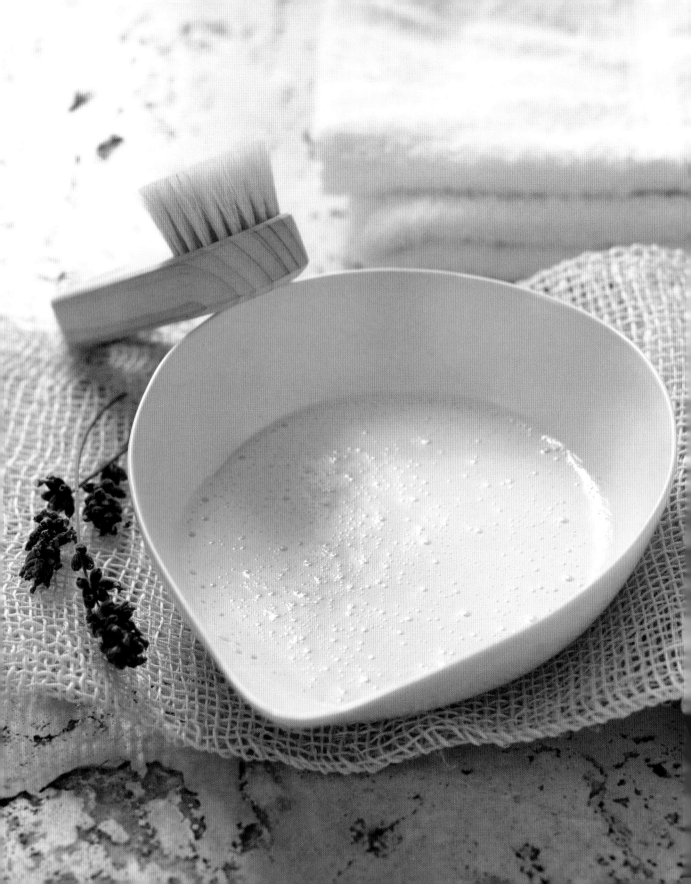

MAKING CLEANSERS

A cleansing routine is essential to support and maintain healthy skin, especially if you live or work in an urban environment with higher levels of pollution. If you have very sensitive skin, test any skin product on a small area of skin first to check that it does not provoke a reaction.

Soothing lavender cleanser

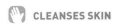 **CLEANSES SKIN**

Makes 60ml (2fl oz)

This is a simple cleanser for sensitive or dry skin. Oats have long been used for their skin-soothing properties, as they are rich in natural polysaccharides that become glutinous in water to create a nurturing wash for delicate skin. Almond oil also soothes and enriches skin, helping to prevent moisture loss, while lavender soothes the skin and adds a gentle fragrance.

INGREDIENTS
25g (scant 1oz) organic oats
a little mineral water
1 egg yolk
3½ tbsp almond oil
5 drops lavender essential oil

METHOD
1 Put the oats in a bowl, pour on enough mineral water to cover, and leave to soak for at least 1 hour.
2 Whisk the egg yolk in a blender or food processor, adding a drop of almond oil at a time. The mixture should be a thick emulsion when all the oil has been added. Add the lavender essential oil, adding a drop at a time so it blends in well.
3 Strain the oats, squeezing all the liquid (oatmilk) into a bowl. Reserve the oatmilk, but discard the oats. Add the oatmilk slowly to the egg mixture, stirring or blending it in gently so that it thins to the consistency of a lotion.
4 Store in a sterilized glass bottle with a tight-fitting lid. Refrigerate and use within 3 days.

Honey and rose petal face scrub

 EXFOLIATES

Makes enough for 1 application

Honey is one of nature's best skin treatments. It softens, soothes, and protects the skin from moisture loss, as well as acting as a lubricant. Rose oil, with its cooling and tonifying properties, and lavender oil, which freshens, and purifies, are also added to this gently exfoliating scrub to help condition and balance the skin and give you a feeling of relaxed well-being.

INGREDIENTS
25g (scant 1oz) dried
   rose petals
2 tbsp dried lavender flowers
1 drop lavender essential oil
1 drop rose essential oil
2 tsp clear honey

METHOD
1 Make an infusion (p.43) using half the rose petals and a cupful of boiling water. Cover and leave to one side.
2 Using a pestle and mortar, grind the remaining rose petals and the lavender flowers until they are of a powdery consistency. Combine the powdered herbs with the essential oils and honey, and add enough rose infusion for the mixture to form a soft paste.
3 To use, apply to the face and gently rub in a circular motion to cleanse the skin.

Lavender and tea tree powder

 SOOTHES SKIN

Makes approx 20g (¾oz)

A cleansing, talc-free, lightly scented body powder such as this is ideal for use before and after sports or strenuous activity to keep skin fresh and to protect against chafing. Apply after bathing to freshly dried skin. Use cotton balls to apply the powder, or just sprinkle it on your body and lightly smooth it over the skin.

INGREDIENTS
20g (¾oz) cornflour
1ml (20 drops) propolis tincture
5 drops lavender essential oil
5 drops tea tree essential oil

METHOD
1 Sift the cornflour evenly onto a wide, flat plate.
2 Mix the propolis tincture and essential oils together and decant into a clean container with a fine mist atomizer.
3 Spray this mix onto the cornflour, taking care to spray evenly and not to saturate the powder, which may cause lumps. Allow the powder to dry.
4 Store the dry powder in an old, clean body powder dispenser or clean pepper shaker. Use within 6 months.

Elderflower and aloe vera facial polish

 EXFOLIATES

Makes enough for 1 treatment

Elderflower is mildly astringent and its anti-inflammatory and emollient properties mean that it has long been beneficial for skin. Combined with cooling aloe vera and soothing chamomile, this gentle, refreshing facial polish is suitable for all skin types. As it contains fresh dairy ingredients, this polish is for immediate use.

INGREDIENTS

25g (scant 1oz) elderflower or
   10 elderflower teabags
25g (scant 1oz) chamomile
   or 10 chamomile teabags
2 tsp aloe vera juice
2 tbsp plain yoghurt

METHOD

1 Make an infusion using 240ml (8fl oz) of boiling water and half the herbs. Cover and leave to one side.
2 Grind the rest of the herbs to a fine powder using a pestle and mortar. If using tea bags, the herbs will already be chopped to a fine powder so they are ready to use.
3 Mix the herbs, aloe vera, and yoghurt, then add the infusion a teaspoon at a time, stirring as you go, until it makes a thin paste (but thick enough not to run off your skin).
4 Apply to the face after cleansing; be sure to avoid the area directly around the eyes and mouth. To exfoliate, gently massage the paste onto your skin with your fingertips in small circular movements.
5 Use the remaining infusion (with extra water as necessary) to rinse off the paste and tone the skin.

Rose body powder

 SOOTHES SKIN

Makes approx 20g (¾oz)

This fragrant, talc-free, floral body powder includes soothing, cooling rose to smooth the skin. Geranium complements and strengthens the scent of rose, while earthy patchouli gives lasting depth. Apply after bathing to freshly dried skin. Use cotton balls to apply the powder, or just sprinkle it on your body and lightly smooth it over the skin.

INGREDIENTS

20g (¾oz) cornflour
5 drops rose absolute essential oil
4 drops geranium essential oil
1 drop patchouli essential oil

METHOD

1 Sift the cornflour evenly onto a wide flat plate.
2 Mix the essential oils together and decant into a clean container with a fine mist atomizer.
3 Spray this mix onto the cornflour, taking care to spray evenly and not to saturate the powder, which may cause lumps.
4 Allow the powder to dry and store in an old, clean body powder dispenser or clean pepper shaker. Use within 6 months.

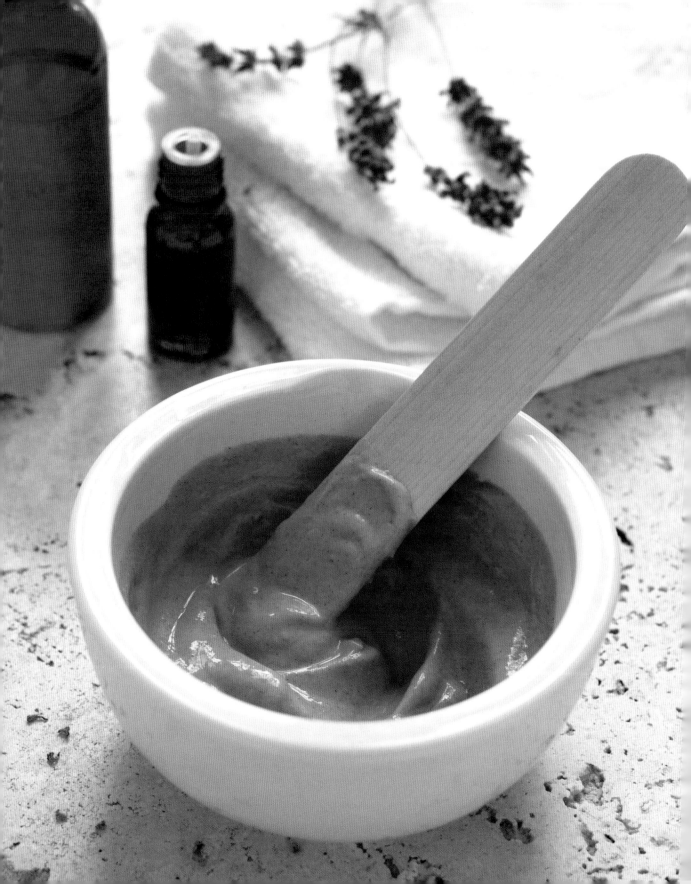

MAKING FACE MASKS

Taking some quiet time to relax with a soothing face pack can be one of life's indulgent pleasures. For extra purification, try a clay mask for a real home spa treat. If you have very sensitive skin, test any skincare product on a small area of skin first to check that it does not provoke a reaction.

Witch hazel and lavender face mask

 CONDITIONS SKIN

Makes enough for 1 treatment

Green clay is the common name for montmorillonite, a naturally occurring mineral-rich clay with highly absorbent properties. As it dries, it draws impurities from the skin and cleanses pores. At the same time, gently astringent witch hazel and soothing lavender tighten the pores and help to promote a clear complexion.

INGREDIENTS
2 tsp green clay powder
2 tsp witch hazel
1 egg, lightly beaten
2 drops lavender essential oil

METHOD
1 Mix the green clay with the witch hazel to make a paste. Add the beaten egg and mix in the lavender essential oil.
2 Apply the pack to your face and leave on for 10 minutes. Gently remove with cool water, then pat dry with a clean towel.

"Spend 10 minutes relaxing with a natural home-made face pack as an indulgent, fragrant treat for your skin and your mind"

Strawberries and cream exfoliating facial mask

 CONDITIONS SKIN

Makes enough for 1 treatment

This fruity mask refreshes and brightens skin. Strawberries, which are rich in natural fruit acids that help to exfoliate the skin, are combined with ground oats to give texture and extra polish, unclog pores, and smooth the skin. As it uses fresh fruit and dairy ingredients, this recipe is for immediate use.

INGREDIENTS
2 tbsp ground oats
3 large ripe strawberries
1 tsp single cream

METHOD
1 Using a pestle and mortar, grind the oats to a fine powder. Mash the strawberries with a fork and combine with the oats. Add the cream and mix to a thick paste (add a little more cream if needed to create the right consistency).
2 Apply the paste to freshly cleansed skin (avoiding the area directly around the eyes and mouth) and leave for 10 minutes.
3 Remove the paste by applying a little water in the palms of your hands to loosen it, then gently rub it away in gentle circular movements. Rinse with cool water and pat dry with a towel.

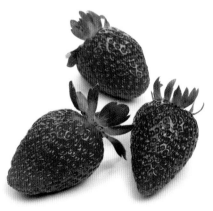

Strawberry (Fragaria x ananassa)
These fresh berries are highly nutritious and full of vitamins. Antioxidant anthocyanins give them their red colour.

Lavender clay mask

 CONDITIONS SKIN

Makes enough for 1–2 treatments

Natural clay minerals draw impurities from the skin and deeply cleanse it. With moisturizing honey and antioxidant-rich aloe vera, and reviving, balancing lavender water and essential oil, this soothing, purifying mask leaves skin feeling fresh and smooth. Store in a sterilized dark glass jar (p.194) with a tight-fitting lid and use within 2 months.

INGREDIENTS
2 tbsp aloe vera juice
1 tsp lavender water
1 tsp clear honey
½ tbsp kaolin powder
1 tbsp bentonite powder
1 drop lavender essential oil

METHOD
1 Combine the aloe vera, lavender water, and honey. Add the clay powders by sprinkling them gradually over the mixed liquids while stirring continually. Press the mixture through a sieve. Add the essential oil and stir again to mix well.
2 Apply to freshly cleansed skin (avoiding the area directly around the eyes and mouth). Leave for 10 minutes. Rinse with warm water and pat dry with a towel.

Grapefruit clay mask

 CONDITIONS SKIN

Makes approx 50ml (1¾fl oz)

This variation on a clay mask is more suited to oilier skin types. Grapefruit is naturally rich in fruit acids, and combined with cleansing clay minerals, mildly astringent and toning witch hazel, and soothing, nutrient-rich aloe vera, it leaves skin cleansed, refreshed, and revitalized. Store in a sterilized dark glass jar with a tight-fitting lid and use within 2 months.

INGREDIENTS
2 tbsp aloe vera juice
1 tsp witch hazel
1 tsp fresh grapefruit juice
1½ tsp kaolin powder
½ tbsp bentonite powder
1 drop lemon essential oil

METHOD
1 Combine the aloe vera juice, witch hazel, and grapefruit juice. Add the clay powders by sprinkling them gradually over the mixed liquids while stirring continually. Press the mixture through a sieve. Add the essential oil and stir again to mix well.
2 Apply to freshly cleansed skin (avoiding the area directly around the eyes and mouth). Leave for 10 minutes. Rinse with warm water and pat dry with a towel.

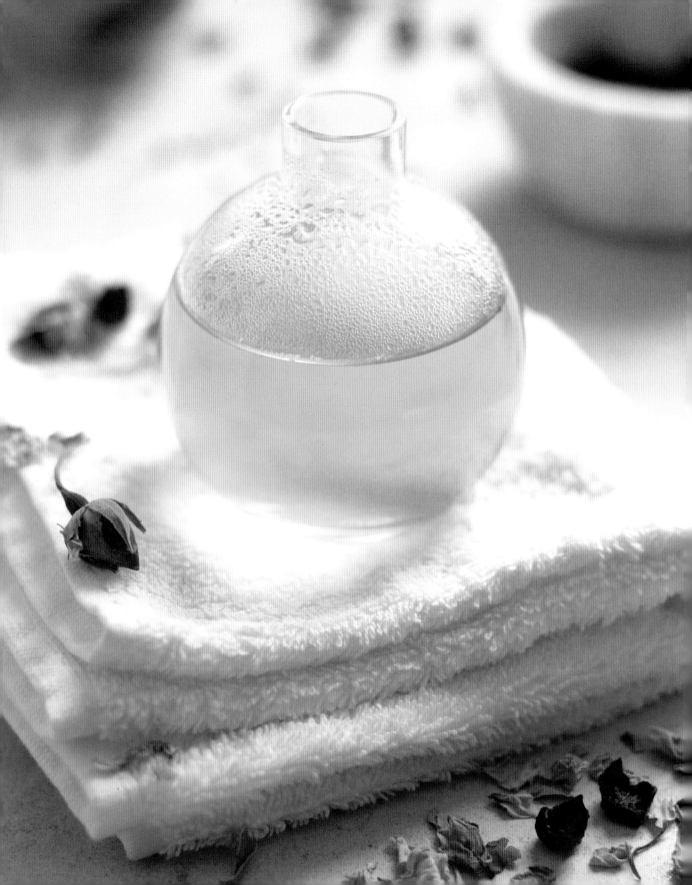

MAKING BATH INFUSIONS

Adding herbs to your bath is one of the easiest and enjoyable ways to benefit from their amazing natural properties. Simply lie back and let the fragrant essences in the infusions lift your spirits, ease any tension headaches, and help you to relax. There's no better way to get a good night's sleep.

Infusions

An infusion is the best way to harness the properties of the softer, green, or flowering parts of a plant. A standard therapeutic infusion is 1 heaped tsp of a single dried herb or 2 tsp of a mixture of dried herbs (for fresh herbs use double the amount) to 175ml (6fl oz) boiling water.

INGREDIENTS
1 heaped tsp dried herb, or 2 tsp chopped fresh herb
175ml (6fl oz) boiling water

METHOD
1 Place the chopped herbs in a cup or teapot, and pour the boiling water over the herbs.
2 Leave to steep for 10 minutes, preferably covered to avoid the loss of volatile oils in the steam. Strain the infusion before use.

Rose and calendula bath infusion

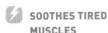 SOOTHES TIRED MUSCLES   RELAXES

Makes enough for 1 bath

This gentle bath infusion nurtures and refreshes, making it a wonderful tonic for dry and sensitive skin. The cooling and balancing properties of roses are renowned; this recipe uses extracts from both the flowers and the vitamin- and flavonoid-rich hips. It also includes cider vinegar to soften the skin and calendula to soothe it.

INGREDIENTS
2 tsp dried rose petals/buds
1 tsp dried rosehips
1 tsp salt
1 tsp cider vinegar
5 drops calendula tincture
8 drops rose essential oil
2 drops geranium essential oil

METHOD
1 Make an infusion (see above) using the rose petals, rosehips, and 500ml (16fl oz) of hot water.
2 Strain the infusion and add the rest of the ingredients.
3 Use immediately by adding to a ready-run warm bath.

Lemon grass and rosemary bath infusion

 RELAXES   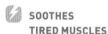 **SOOTHES TIRED MUSCLES**

Makes enough for 1 bath

Lemon grass, bay, and rosemary are all herbs that are well known for their fragrant, culinary use, but they can be just as useful in body care. This stimulating and warming aromatic bath blend eases tired muscles and is ideal for restoring the body after physical activity, sport, or periods of over-exertion.

INGREDIENTS

2 tsp dried bay leaves, chopped
1 tsp dried rosemary
5 drops lemon grass essential oil

METHOD

Make an infusion (p.43) with 500ml (16fl oz) of water, the bay leaves, and the rosemary. When cooled, add the lemon grass essential oil. Use immediately, adding it to a freshly run bath.

Lavender and aloe vera bath infusion

 RELAXES   **SOOTHES TIRED MUSCLES**

Makes enough for 1 bath

This bath infusion will soothe sensitive skin and encourage a sense of well-being and relaxation. Lavender, which initially has a reviving, restorative effect, has been long used to ease both body and mind. This makes it a perfect remedy in this gentle bath blend, along with soothing aloe vera and nurturing chamomile.

INGREDIENTS

2 tsp lavender
2 tsp chamomile
30ml (2 tbsp) aloe vera juice
10 drops lavender essential oil

METHOD

1 Make an infusion (p.43) with 500ml (16fl oz) of water and the lavender and chamomile flowers. When cooled, add the aloe vera juice and lavender essential oil.
2 Use immediately, adding it to a freshly run bath. Ensure that your bath is not too hot if you have dry or sensitive skin.

Seaweed and arnica bath infusion

 RELAXES

SOOTHES
TIRED MUSCLES

Makes enough for 1 bath

This revitalizing blend restores the body after a long day. Nutrient-rich bladderwrack seaweed is traditionally used to soothe irritated and inflamed tissues in the body, and here it is partnered with arnica – a famous remedy for bumps, bruises, and strains – and a stimulating blend of essential oils. Add to your bath water, lie back, and relax.

INGREDIENTS

½ tsp bladderwrack
1 tsp comfrey
2 tsp juniper berries
2 heaped tsp sea salt
5 drops arnica tincture
2 drops pine oil
2 drops lavender essential oil
2 drops lemon essential oil
2 drops juniper essential oil

METHOD

1 Make an infusion (p.43) with 500ml (16fl oz) of water and the dried herbs.
2 Add the salt and stir until well dissolved. Mix in the arnica tincture and the essential oils.
3 Use immediately, adding the infusion to a freshly run bath.

Detox bath infusion

 STIMULATES
CIRCULATION

 SOOTHES
TIRED MUSCLES

Makes enough for 1 bath

To encourage the elimination of toxins from the body, nutrient-rich bladderwrack is combined with cleansing sea salt, circulation-boosting juniper, black pepper, and lemon essential oils. For the best results, try dry body brushing with a natural bristle brush or body mitt before your bath to exfoliate the skin and energize the body.

INGREDIENTS

½ tsp bladderwrack
1 tsp celery seeds
2 tsp fennel seeds
2 heaped tsp sea salt
2 drops juniper essential oil
2 drops black pepper essential oil
2 drops lemon essential oil
2 drops eucalyptus essential oil

METHOD

Make an infusion (p.43) with 500ml (16fl oz) of water and the dried herbs. Add the essential oils to the salt, then add the salt to the infusion and stir until well dissolved. Use immediately, adding it to a freshly run bath.

Fennel seed (*Foeniculum vulgare*)
These seeds are actually small, strongly flavoured, aromatic fruits, which make a cleansing, toning infusion for the skin.

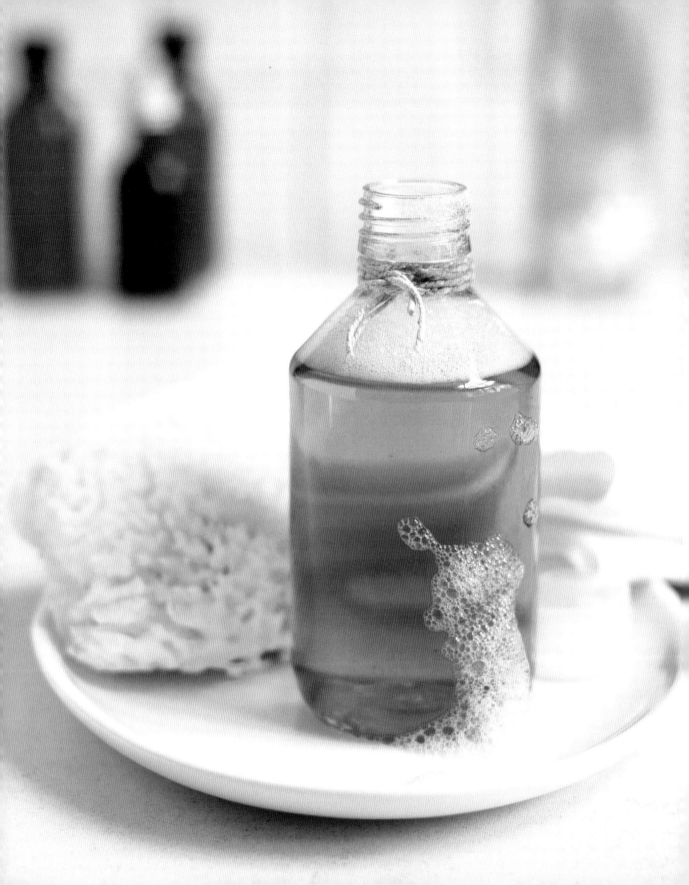

MAKING HAIR AND SCALP TREATMENTS

Beautiful hair depends on a healthy scalp. Keep your scalp in good condition by washing your hair in warm, not hot, water, and using home-made herbal treatments to add extra nutrition. Then rinse through for shiny, revitalized hair with bounce.

Comfrey hair tonic

 TREATS ALL HAIR TYPES

INGREDIENTS
3 tsp dried calendula
3 tsp dried comfrey
1 tsp dried horsetail

Makes 1 treatment

Comfrey has a conditioning effect on the hair and scalp, as it is rich in an extract, allantoin, that helps to encourage natural cellular regeneration. Calendula soothes the scalp and is an excellent rinse for hair alongside shine-enhancing horsetail. This simple tonic nourishes both the hair and scalp to restore your hair's natural vitality.

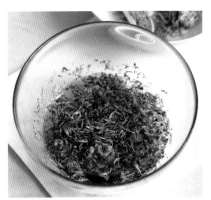

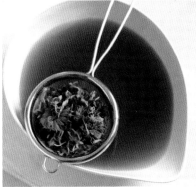

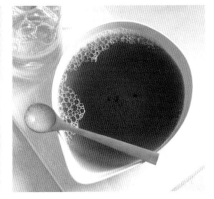

1 *Infuse the dried herbs* with 100ml (3fl oz) of boiling water in a bowl.

2 *Allow to stand* and cool for 20 minutes, then strain through a sieve into a bowl. Discard the herbs.

3 *Add the strained liquid* to your shampoo up to a maximum ratio of 50 per cent (the more you add, the thinner the shampoo will be). Use any excess infusion as a final rinse for the hair.

Acknowledgments

Neal's Yard Remedies would like to thank the following for their valuable contribution to making this book happen: Julie Wood, Elly Phillips, Dr Pauline Hili and the NYR technical team past and present, and Dr Merlin Willcox.

Dorling Kindersley would like to thank the team at Neal's Yard Remedies, Peacemarsh, for the use of the organic physic garden in July and August 2010 for many of the herb photographs in this book. We would also like to thank Philip Robbshow at Sheepdrove Organic Farm for his help.

Thanks to the following for supplying plants for photography: Arne Herbs, Jekka's Herb Farm, Petersham Nurseries, Poyntzfield Herb Nursery, and South Devon Chilli Farm.

Illustrations Debbie Maizels
Art direction Luis Peral, Nicky Collings
Food styling Jane Lawrie
Prop styling Wei Tang
Proofreading Jennifer Latham
Recipe testing Katy Greenwood
Editorial assistance Roxanne Benson-Mackey, Kajal Mistry
Design assistance Danaya Bunnag, Emma Forge
DK Picture Library Lucy Claxton, Romaine Werblow

The Authors

Susan Curtis
Susan runs a busy practice as a homeopath and naturopath and is the Director of Natural Health for Neal's Yard Remedies. She is the author of several books, including Essential Oils, and co-author of Natural Healing for Women. Susan has two children and is passionate about helping people to live a more natural and healthy lifestyle.

Louise Green
An avid supporter of the organic movement and eco-living, Louise has spent 15 years at Neal's Yard Remedies in a variety of roles ranging from buying to product development, and most recently as Head of Sustainability. Louise lives in London and is expecting her first child.

Penelope Ody MNIMH
Penelope qualified as a medical herbalist in the 1980s and practised as a consultant herbalist for 12 years. Since then she has written more than 20 books on both Western and Chinese herbalism and runs workshops on traditional uses of culinary and medicinal herbs at her home in Hampshire.

Dragana Vilinac
A fourth-generation herbalist widely respected for her vast knowledge and expertise, Dragana's passion for herbal medicine has taken her around the world, and has led her to train in disciplines including Western Herbal Medicine and Traditional Chinese Medicine. Dragana is Head Herbalist for Neal's Yard Remedies.